The Power of Protein for Weight Loss

Accelerate Weight Loss With Protein

RON KNESS

Contents

Disclaimer

This publication is for informational purposes only and is not intended as medical advice. Medical advice should always be obtained from a qualified medical professional for any health conditions or symptoms associated with them.

Every possible effort has been made in preparing and researching this material. We make no warranties with respect to the accuracy, applicability of its contents or any omissions.

See your healthcare professional before starting any diet or exercise program!

The Power of Protein

Anyone who has ever tried to lose weight knows that there are ups and downs, ebbs and flows. Some people get frustrated and stop trying to lose weight because they go on these complicated diets that either introduce foods that are as appetizing as cardboard or they strictly limit foods they love.

Not only is that not appealing and not healthy for the body, but it doesn't lead to long term, successful weight loss. One of the simplest ways to lose weight is to make sure you're getting the protein that your body needs.

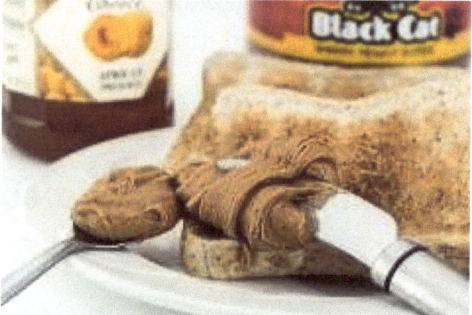

If you're eliminating or severely limiting protein, or simply not paying attention to the fact that you're loading up on carbs and ignoring the protein aspect, then it could be one of the reasons why your weight loss journey has been a struggle.

Eating Protein Leads to Energy

Your body was made to need protein. You need it from head to toe. The cells throughout your body have to have it. Without enough protein, you'll end up with thinning hair and weak nails.

Your body will struggle to stay healthy - to keep your muscles and tissues in good working order. You'll suffer from a lack of certain hormones and you can damage your bones without having enough protein in your diet.

But a huge reason that you need to eat protein might surprise you. You need protein because it gives you energy. And energy is what enables you to be able to do whatever it is that you need to do throughout the day.

Lack of protein is a big reason why so many diets people have tried, fail. Who cares what foods you eat when you're so tired and so drained that all you want to do is collapse on the sofa and not move?

Diets that don't include a focus on protein will eventually wear you out and you won't want to stick to them. And you shouldn't. You need protein to give you the right amount of energy that will sustain you all the way through your journey to weight loss success.

With the right amount of protein, you'll get a boost in your energy supply - and that will carry you through your day to day activities. When you have more energy, you end up feeling better emotionally and physically.

You'll be surprised at how much more you can accomplish when your body has a solid energy supply. How protein helps to provide you with this energy is by stabilizing your system.

Certain sugary, carb-loaded foods will give you quick bursts of energy that make you feel like you can run all day for a few minutes - but they inevitably lead to crashes where you feel more drained than before.

Protein works to make sure that the amount of glucose in your system doesn't have those high peaks and lows. It works to keep your blood sugar steadier, which in turn leads to a steady amount of energy all day long.

You might have been on low protein diets in the past that made you realize that not only did you not lose weight, but you felt like you were dragging yourself just to be able to function.

When you feel like that, it's your body's way of letting you know that it needs something it's lacking. What happens when you don't get enough protein is you'll find yourself struggling with cognitive function once your energy level drops.

Your brain can't function the way that it's meant to without the amino acids from proteins. Many people who are trying to lose weight experience this struggle with cognitive function, not realizing it's caused by not having the right amount of protein.

It can push you to make impulsive decisions. For example, when they crash because they don't have enough energy, they immediately seek something that's loaded with carbs to try to jumpstart themselves again.

Some people don't get enough protein and try to use other things in its place, like high energy drinks or caffeine. But when the effects of those wear off, then you end up feeling more fatigued than before.

Protein in Your Diet Can Help You Lose Weight

Wanting to lose weight is something that many people are familiar with. Those extra pounds can happen for a variety of reasons. While losing weight doesn't happen overnight, it's not as difficult as you think as long as the steps you're taking to try to lose aren't counterproductive.

You'll want to stay away from fad diet eating plans and any advice that calls on you to put your body at any kind of nutritional risk.

Some of the risks associated with diets include ones that want to eliminate certain foods such as protein.

One of the biggest mistakes that you can make when you're trying to lose weight is not having enough protein with your meals. Many people know some of the more widely reported foods that help with weight loss, but don't know that protein foods are the best ones to help with a diet.

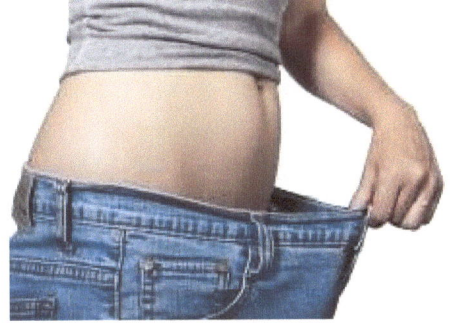

There's a good reason for this. You know how you eat a meal when you're dieting and then two hours later all of a sudden you feel as if you haven't eaten in days?

That's what happens when you don't get enough protein. Protein stops hunger in its tracks. It can do this because protein foods don't digest quickly like other foods do.

It sticks around in your system longer, so you end up not feeling hungry for longer periods of time. When you're not hungry as often, it cuts down on those in between meal cravings that inevitably lead to weight loss sabotage.

These snack cravings are caused by eating foods that don't have enough nutritional value like protein does. Because your hunger is satisfied longer when you have protein, you won't be eating as many calories throughout the day, which will also help fuel weight loss.

Also, when you have plenty of protein in your diet, you're not dealing with the steep energy lows that drive people to grab whatever is handy to eat. Getting the shakes and feeling weak has led to some people consuming as much as an entire day's worth of calories in one hunger fueled binge.

Since you'll feel full longer, you'll be able to better manage how you eat once you do feel hungry. More good news about making sure you eat protein for weight loss is that consuming it helps propel weight loss.

There are certain foods that, you once you eat them, run through your digestive system with very little effort involved in digesting them. But protein foods put your body to work during the digestive process, known as the "thermal effect". Because of the thermal effect, your net calories is much lower due to the number of calories it took just to break down the protein you ate.

Because of that, your body is burning calories at a longer and higher rate to digest meals containing protein than ones that don't. So in effect, the simple act of eating is spurring on weight loss.

You'll often see weight loss talked about in conjunction with fat burning. Your body can naturally burn fat, but not unless it has what it needs. Without enough protein, your body can't burn fat.

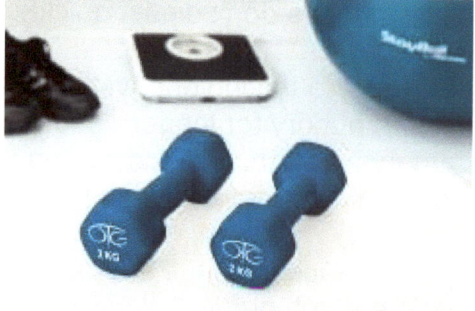

There's a good reason for this. When you move around and go about your day, your body uses energy. It takes this energy from the foods that you consume. When you don't have the type of foods that work to protect your lean muscles, then what happens is your body will lose muscle.

And that's something that you don't want. In order to protect your body from burning muscle rather than fat stores, it has to have protein. You want it to tap into the right source for energy.

Protein Can Help You with Getting Lean

Protein comes in a variety of foods and some of it contains more grams than other types of foods. However you get your protein, it's important that you are getting enough if you're trying to lose weight.

Protein speeds up the process of burning calories, it works to help keep you healthy and it builds muscles. It's the type of food that you need on a daily basis when you want to burn fat and shed pounds.

But with all of the different diet advice on the market now, knowing how much and when to eat protein isn't easy to figure out. You have to consume what your body needs and if the consumption of protein is out of balance, it can make losing weight more difficult.

You want to know exactly how much protein to have in your diet. Your muscles need protein in order to keep your metabolism higher. Without it, you won't burn calories as fast because your muscles won't have what they need.

So what's a good rule of thumb to have when it comes to eating protein for the purpose of losing weight? Your current weight and how much you move or exercise is what you need to go by to figure how much protein you need to have.

For people who work out heavily and have a focus on wanting to build muscle, you'll need more protein than someone who wants to lose weight and doesn't plan on building muscle.

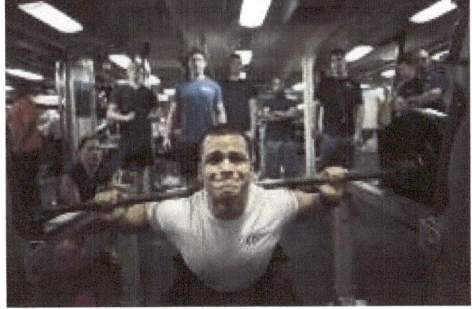

The more active you are every day as well as the harder you work out, the more protein you'll need to eat. Someone who's trying to lose weight and has a light activity level won't need as much for their body as someone who has a harder, more intense activity level.

Getting lean means that you should eat plenty of protein - but not all at once in big, heavy meals. Instead, you need to spread out the protein consumption throughout your day.

This means eating protein five or six times a day versus having protein over the course of three meals a day. You want the protein to keep your glucose steady so that it keeps hunger at bay.

Plus, when you eat protein more often than three times a day, you tend to eat less than if you only had it three times a day. What this does is help you keep down the caloric intake as well as pushes your body to keep your metabolism up.

The basic recommended daily intake of protein is 46 grams for women and 56 grams for men. That number goes up, based on whether or not you're attempting to build muscle mass while losing weight.

If you are, then you would base your grams of protein according to how much you weigh. You can find calculators and nutritional trackers online to help you meet your goals.

The Benefits of Protein During Weight Loss

By now, you already know that protein helps keep you feeling fuller, longer so that you're not tempted to overeat and hinder your weight loss efforts. You also know that it helps your metabolism to stay in high gear.

But there's a lot more that eating protein can do for you to help you be successful. Even carrying an extra ten pounds of weight can make you feel fatigued and can impact your muscle mass.

Because most people who do desire to lose weight don't always eat the healthiest, they don't get the daily recommended amount of protein. So they feel fatigued and experience a loss in muscle mass due to the deficit in their protein intake.

Once you correct that and make eating enough protein a priority, the fatigue will go away and you'll see a difference in your muscle mass. People who are overweight - even by as little as twenty pounds - put themselves at risk for developing diseases like diabetes.

Making sure that your blood sugar levels don't go through extreme ups and downs is one of the key ways to keep from developing weight gain related diabetes.

When it comes to trying to lose weight, there's a side to it that a lot of people don't often take into consideration. That's the emotional element. Sure, people do get upset when weight loss efforts don't seem to pay off - but there could be another reason to explain why you just feel a little off.

Maybe you feel a little down or more irritable than you used to be. One of the reasons that you may be experiencing problems with mood stabilization is due to not having protein in your diet.

Protein is known to not only stabilize your moods but it can also boost them. The amino acids in proteins are needed for your nervous system to be able to work correctly.

It's also needed to help your body process the production of hormones, which impact your mood and energy. A lack of protein can make it harder to concentrate and can affect your mood to the point where you'll get frustrated easier and feel irritable.

This can push you to overeat or make bad food choices. When your body has enough protein, it aids in the production of hormones that cause calmness and give you a better ability to cope with stress.

You'll even get a good night's sleep when you eat enough protein. The right amount of protein consumption works within your body to get rid of insomnia and boost your ability to fall asleep naturally.

All of these benefits given to you by protein work to not only help you take off the extra weight, but to maintain that loss for the long haul. The best formula for protein intake will depend on your goals and how you feel, since everyone is unique in their nutritional reactions.

Dietary Changes to Maximize the Use of Protein

Anytime that you're trying to lose weight, you need to make sure you're getting the protein that helps you reach your goals. The best way to do that is by maximizing the use of protein in your meal plan.

Protein and Carbs

It's a given that you need both protein and carbs as part of any healthy plan to lose weight. But it's not going to do you any good to make sure you're getting plenty of protein if you're still not paying close attention to the amount of carbs that you eat.

You have to eat fewer carbs, but up your intake of protein to create the balance that your body needs. Some people who are trying to shed unwanted pounds think that because protein is necessary for muscles and tissue repair and does all sorts of good things for the 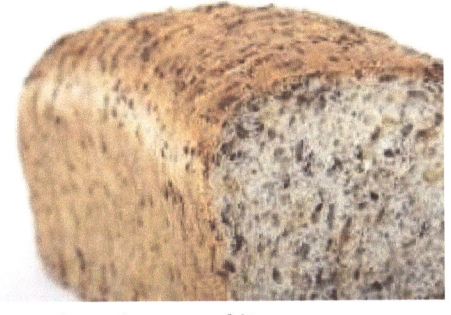 body, that you need to have an abundance of it.

Your body can't use large influxes of protein all at one time to aid in weight loss. You can certainly eat it, but the weight loss benefit you hoped to gain from larger portions of protein won't happen.

That's because your body has to digest the protein in order for it to be able to use it. You can't absorb a lot of it at once, so that's why you should forget eating the larger meals with all of the carbs and protein and eat smaller meals instead.

Eat your protein in increments of 5-7 times a day. You can do that in the form of three light meals and two snacks – one in the morning and another in the afternoon. If you do that, your body is better able to absorb it and it will help you lose weight. Some diet plans will tell you that the more protein you eat, or if you focus solely on eating protein, then you'll lose weight faster.

But you're wasting your effort because your body uses the protein that you eat based on your body weight. What happens when you don't eat fewer carbs and you don't balance your protein is that your body has a cut off limit for what it will process and use.

Both extra carbs and protein that your body doesn't need goes exactly where you don't want it to go – it turns into fat. A quarter to half of all of your calories should be protein. A good starting point is 50% carbohydrates, 30% protein and 20% fat. Then you can adjust from there depending on the results you are seeing.

The thing about losing weight is that you really do need to be flexible with how you plan your eating. Not every day of your life is the same. You might use more energy on one day while barely using any the next.

You can adjust your carb intake based on what goes on in your life. When you're having some really strenuous workout days where you're pushing yourself, you can and should have more carbs on those days - but not so much that it's counterproductive to weight loss.

Protein and Carbs: How Much Do You Need?

Protein is key to losing weight. You need to stay healthy, you need your muscles to be strong and you need plenty of energy if you're adding exercise to your routine.

Eating protein throughout the day will keep your metabolism up as well as your energy. You also get your energy from carbs. But there are some carbs that don't offer you much in the way of health benefits.

These empty carbs will raise your sugar level, give you a fast burst of energy, then drain it all away. These roller-coaster ups and downs aren't good for you and can derail your weight loss plans.

That's why it's important for you to know exactly how much
protein you need and how many carbs you should be consuming. When it comes to eating for weight loss, most people struggle to get in the amount of protein they need while getting in too many carbs.

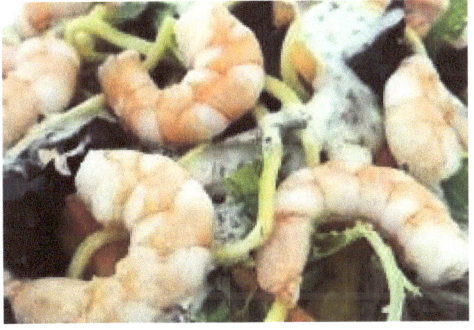

This out of balance eating not only causes weight gain, but also fatigue. Knowing how much protein you should eat is a fairly easy fix. You need approximately 0.8 grams for every kilogram of weight.

If you break that down, it's between 40-50 grams of protein for women who are not active and 50-60 grams for men who aren't active. These numbers change once you add an exercise program.

When it comes to knowing how much you need to eat in the carbohydrate category, you need to know that it's best to use a standard or average suggestion.

Obviously, to lose weight, you would need to eat fewer carbs than what you have been eating. When you're figuring up the amount of carbs you need, always figure out your activity level first.

Then apply your age and your weight. Most eating plans suggests a carb level of between 50 and 100 grams per day when you're trying to lose weight. You need to listen to your body once you have a calculation in mind.

It will tell you whether or not you're eating enough carbs. If you're watching your carb level intake and keeping it lower than you usually have, you can sometimes experience side effects.

Some of the more well know side effects of not eating enough carbs are nausea, headaches, shakes, bad breath, no energy, irritability and constipation. You can also experience low blood sugar levels that leave you feeling weak and dizzy.

One thing to keep in mind is that you can add more protein to your diet when you cut back on processed carbs. You can easily do that by cutting way down or better yet, eliminating the junk food from your day.

Convenience Eating

Elaborate, time consuming meals and snacks are a thing of the past. Today, it's all about convenience. This isn't necessarily a bad thing. Getting to eat your food fast can be a time saver that gives you more time to do the things that you want to do.

Plus, it can be an energy saver. No one wants to spend two or three hours working on a meal. The faster the better has become the norm. However, there can be a price to pay for convenience.

Not all quick foods are good for you. They can be loaded with calories, carbs and sodium - none of which are helpful to your body in excess.

But when you're trying to lose weight, you need to play for convenience because there will be those days when you're going to have to grab something to eat faster than you expected.

If you're not prepared, one of two things will happen. You'll snack while you're waiting for your food to get ready and can easily add an extra 300 or more calories to your daily intake.

Or, you'll end up stressed and hungry at a fast food or other type of restaurant and you'll end up overeating. Convenience doesn't have to mean foods that are bad for you or foods that you end up going through a drive-through to get.

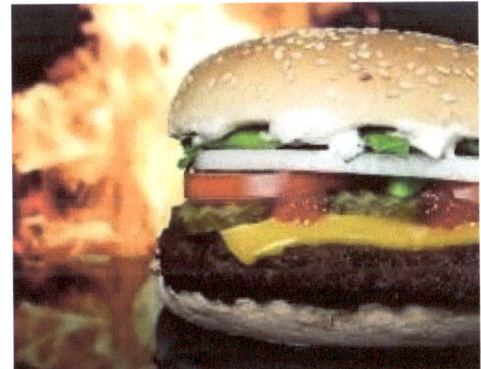

You can plan ahead and make sure that your meals - as well as your snacks - are readily available. You can balance them out with the right amount of protein and minerals.

One way to do that is to have a way to keep food that's fast and accessible on hand. Obviously, if you need some protein fast, you might not have time to wait for some lean meat to cook.

You certainly don't want to eat something that's processed to get the protein. But there is something that you can do. Make sure that you have foods on hand for weight loss that are well known for their convenience.

This would be foods like protein shakes that are already prepared. These will boost your energy without giving you the crash of energy you want to avoid. Plus, they're good for you.

They come in a variety and you can pick them up in cans, bottles or use the powder to quickly make your own right at home. There are also convenience bars you can get.

You can get protein bars that contain all of the protein that you need for a snack or even a meal. It's important (not just for your weight loss but for your overall health) that you plan your meals for convenience.

When you know what you're going to eat for your meals and what your snack options are, it makes it easier for you to make the right choices. Plus, there are steps that you can take that can help you stay on top of making sure you're getting the right levels of protein as well as carbs.

You can also make sure that you're getting all of your nutritional needs met by simply planning. The best way to do that is to get a calendar that has the larger squares on it.

These should give you plenty of space to write in. Then what you do is write out the meal that you're having for each day of the week. You would do this for each meal and divide the meals by at least five so you spread out the protein intake.

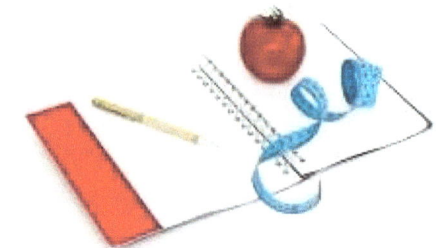

Beside each of the meals that you write out, you would list a P followed by a short dash to indicate the grams of protein you're getting. So your calendar might look something like P-10.

For carbs, you would use a C. This is a quick-glance way of you being able to track your protein and keep your weight loss goals on track. For your snacks, you would list those and use the same letters. For weight loss, your calories consumed should be around 500 calories less than you burned. That will result in a one pound loss of weight per week which is a good sustainable loss.

The key to great meal planning is to stay organized and buy foods that support your weight loss decisions. If it's not in the house, you can't eat it. Or, learn how to eat small, mindful portions and pair a protein with a carb to stay satisfied, longer.

Ten Tips for You to Use to Help Maximize Protein Every Day

When you talk about protein and how it helps the body with weight and muscles, some people get a mental image of a bodybuilder with both hands loaded with meat.

You don't have to constantly walk around with protein in hand in order to add it to your diet. Making sure that you get the amount of protein that you need is a lot easier than you can imagine.

#1. Make sure that you're not substituting filler protein for the real deal.

You can buy protein in convenience packaging. But some of these meals don't give you the full weight of the protein. Instead, extenders, binders or fillers are used.

Some of these are products that aren't in any way associated with healthy protein. So you don't get the true amount of protein that you think you're getting. You want real, lean protein options.

#2. Make sure that you're eating protein in some form with every meal.

This will help make sure that you're getting an amount of protein that's helpful with weight loss. Plus, you'll stay fuller - which will also help you lose weight. So if you know you're eating a piece of fruit, which is a carb, add a chunk of cheese or lean meat to go with it.

#3. Seek out ways to increase the amount of protein in each meal.

When it comes to protein, many people who want to lose weight end up concentrating on the main entrée as their only source of it. You should look for ways with each meal to up your intake of protein.

That means you need to look for how you can add it to your side dishes and any appetizers. For example, if you were eating a low carb tortilla filled with refried beans and cheese, you could put fewer beans and add lean grilled chicken to the burrito.

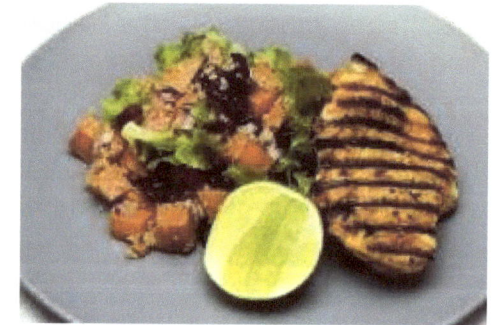

#4. Make snack time synonymous with protein.

Every time you have a snack, it should include some type of protein. You'll get the benefits of an energy boost along with soothing any munchies that you might be experiencing.

#5. Consider other forms of protein.

Some people, especially those who aren't juicers and don't use protein supplements, don't realize that not all protein has to be eaten. Adding protein to beverages is a quick and easy way of adding protein to your meals or snacks.

#6. Become a meal prepper or planner.

Planning your meals can help you see if your carbs are taking over your proteins. By cutting back on the carbohydrates, you'll have room in your stomach for more protein.

#7. Ditch junk food for good.

Weight loss tips always tell you to cut out the junk food. It's not just because these foods are high in empty calories and not healthy. It's because they take up room in your calorie and carb intake that you can use for protein.

#8. To make sure that you're getting the protein that you need and keeping the cravings for junk food at bay, keep some with you.

There are convenience protein snacks that you can put in your car for those times when you're stuck in traffic and dying to have something to eat. You can also take protein foods to the office with you every day and keep some at your desk. This way, you're not tempted to get up and hit the vending machine when you're feeling hungry.

#9. Eat on a schedule.

Protein can help you lose weight more effectively when you're eating your meals and your snacks at the same time every day. This keeps your body's energy levels up and allows you to be more mindful with your meals.

#10. Remember that not every protein is equal.

The amino acids in protein do vary from food to food and so do the grams of protein. To make sure that you're not eating too many calories all day long, choose foods that have more grams of protein.

The Best Meat Proteins for Your Body

There are dozens of reasons that you need to eat meat and all of them end up being because they're good for your overall health. The protein in meat is used to keep your bones and muscles strong and it's also used in hormone production.

Meat proteins also help you lose weight while keeping your energy level up at the same time. There are many forms of meat, and some are more beneficial to your body than others.

Beef

Beef is a well-known source of protein. This red meat is also packed full of iron as well, and depending on what type of beef you eat and how you prepare it, it can be extremely good for your body.

One of the reasons to consider making sure you consume meals containing beef in your eating plan is because the iron level in it is higher than that contained in poultry or seafood.

This is important because surprisingly, many adults don't get enough daily iron intake - which affects their ability to lose weight. A lack of protein will cause a deterioration in concentration and increase fatigue, sabotaging your plans to work out.

Along with the different types of beef, you'll encounter different levels of fat in this meat. That's what you have to watch out for. You want the protein benefit, but you don't want the fat content.

This is why you should always choose the leanest cuts of meats for your meals. Most people shy away from red meat when they're trying to lose weight. They believe that the meat is too high in fat content to be good for them when dieting.

But the truth is, when you choose red meat that's lean, the fat content isn't that high. For example, you can choose to broil a serving of ground beef. If you choose the one that's 90% or more lean for a 3 ounce serving, then you get about 200 calories with 22 grams of protein and only 10 grams of fat.

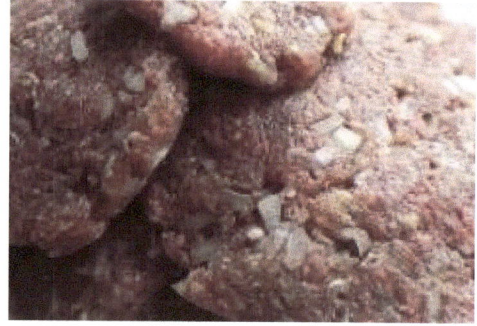

The leaner the meat cut, the lower the grams of fat will be. If you choose to have a steak, you just want to pay attention to how much marbling the meat cut has. This is the fat in the meat and it also tells you how tender that meat will turn out to be once cooked.

The beef that has the most fat is usually labeled as a prime cut. When choosing beef cuts such as steaks, look for ones that are labeled USDA Select. This is the cut that has the least amount of fat in it, but you still get a good amount of protein.

Not only should you pay attention to the amount of marbling when choosing a steak, but do the same when you're planning on making a roast or some ribs.

If you're planning on grilling some burgers for a meal, you won't see the marbling - which is why you have to rely on the fat percentage on the label.

Lean beef is packed with protein, vitamins and 8 essential amino acids so it's a good choice when picking out meat for your meals. You can even buy lean steaks like filet mignon and have the butcher grind it into beef patties for you if you want something really lean.

Pork

Strangely, most people don't associate pork with protein or weight loss. But that's because it's gotten an unfair reputation as being the kind of meat that's not healthy for people to eat.

This is a myth. This myth exists because when pork is talked about, people immediately think of bologna or sausage or bacon. It's true that those foods aren't healthy for you to consume in large quantities and they're loaded with fat as well as sodium.

The right cut of pork is actually very good for you. Not only is it white meat, which is healthier to eat, but it's loaded with protein that can help you on your weight loss journey.

Certain types of pork contain as much protein as beef does and it's equally healthy. When shopping for pork cuts, remember to choose the ones that have loin as part of the label.

These are the best cuts of the meat and they're also leaner. What you want to do is to look for ones with labels like pork chops, pork loin and pork tenderloin. Not only are they loaded with protein, but they also don't have as many calories as you might have thought.

Many people who are trying to lose weight will choose pork tenderloin. When compared to beef cuts, not only is it lower in fat content in many instances, but it's also lower in price.

It's a lean meat that's easy to make and tastes delicious. When you compare pork tenderloin to a 3 ounce serving of ground beef, not only does the tenderloin have the same amount of protein, but it only has about 3 grams of fat compared to 10.

The meat can be grilled or roasted just like a steak can. Plus, besides the great taste and the protein it contains that will help you lose weight, you can enjoy all of the healthy vitamins and minerals it contains.

Pork is loaded with them. It has iron and phosphorus as well as thiamin and selenium, zinc and a plenty of the B vitamins as well. This helps your body run smoothly, giving you energy and vitality to pursue your weight loss.

Poultry

When you think of poultry, usually the first meat that comes to mind is chicken. That's because this meat is one of the most popular ones you'll find in this category thanks to the amount of protein it contains.

There is a good, healthy way to prepare chicken that will give you vitamins, minerals and the protein that will help you to be able to lose weight. Of all the parts of chicken to choose to eat, the breast meat has the least amount of fat.

It also has the most protein. As long as you cook the chicken using one of the healthier methods, it will help your weight loss efforts. However, if you cook chicken the wrong way, you can pile on the fat as well as the calories.

If you fry chicken in a heavily saturated oil, it's not as good for you as if it were prepared other ways. Frying is one of the most often used methods for making chicken.

But fried chicken is one of the worst ways to prepare this meat because of how high the fat and calorie level rises. Eating chicken this way or consuming spicy chicken wings or other flavors in chicken wings is high in saturated fat and calories.

You'll still get the protein, but you'll be hindering your weight loss. Chicken is a popular source of protein because if it's prepared properly, it can be a low-calorie, low-sodium meal.

It can be eaten for all of your meals and if cubed, is also a great snack to have. To get the most benefit from the protein in chicken without the fat and calories, choose the white cuts over the dark ones.

Chicken breasts are a good option, but make sure that you remove all of the skin before you eat it. In case you're wondering how chicken compares to beef when it comes to the amount of protein it has, one cup of chicken breasts cubed has about 5 grams of fat and a more than 40 grams of protein.

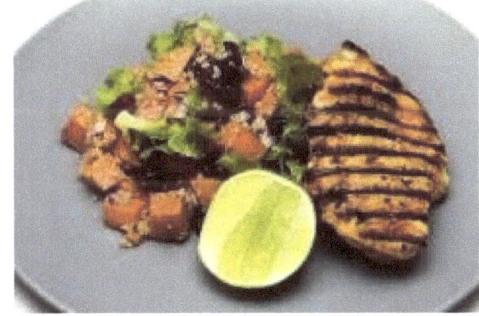

Even a small drumstick on a chicken has a high amount of protein. One of them alone has 23 grams of it. Turkey is another popular meat in the poultry category that's loaded with protein.

Not everyone cooks with turkey and they're really missing out on the high amount of protein contained in this meat.

One pound of turkey contains an astonishing 133 grams of protein.

It's one of the most often chosen meats during the holidays, but you can get all of the weight loss effects from the protein by making sure you have turkey added to dishes every week.

Substituting lean ground turkey for lean ground beef can give you a great serving of protein. Plus, it's packed with vitamins and minerals. It's the kind of meat that helps you build your muscles if that's part of your exercise plan.

Building lean muscle by using protein causes you to lose weight because a higher muscle mass burns calories more efficiently. Plus, turkey is rich in tryptophan, an amino acid.

You need this in order for your brain to produce serotonin, which boosts your mood. So if you're someone who's an emotional eater, you might want to choose turkey as the protein that you eat more often.

By choosing turkey as your protein, it will help you resist the temptation to give in to feeding your emotions. While it's not as popular as chicken or turkey, another type of poultry food that's loaded with protein is duck.

A serving of this meat contains 27 grams of protein. Though it tastes delicious, one of the problems with getting your protein allowance from duck is that this type of meat can be very fatty if made with the skin on.

But if you take off the skin before you eat it, then you gain the protein benefits without the high fat content. Again, it's all in preparation and how you consume it that determines whether it's beneficial to your goals or not.

Another option is to eat eggs. If there's one protein food that's received a bad rap over the years, it's eggs in any form that you make them. Many nutritional experts came back years after telling people to limit their egg intake because eggs were supposedly bad for your cholesterol and admitted they were wrong.

Eggs are far from being a food that's bad for you. In fact, it's the opposite. This natural food is so great for your body that it can prevent many diseases and health conditions that other foods can't help you with.

Eggs are full of vitamins and minerals. They contain a lot of the important B vitamins as well as vitamin A. They're also packed with nutrients like phosphorus, folate and selenium.

They also have many of the trace elements that are good for your body. One of the erroneous warnings about eggs had to do with the way that they supposedly raised the cholesterol levels.

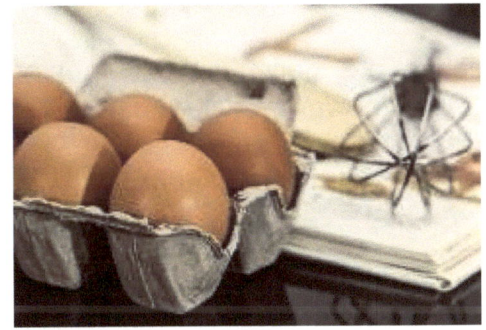

But new studies found that the prior warnings about linking eggs to high cholesterol levels were wrong. And the amount of fat in an egg is actually small. It contains 5 grams of fat, but it's not the kind of fat that's bad for your heart.

Your body naturally makes cholesterol itself. In some people, there's a higher cholesterol production than in other people, and this can contribute to bad cholesterol numbers being higher than they should.

Eggs are low in calories. A large egg has about 70 calories, which makes it the perfect choice when you want to add protein as part of a healthy way to lose weight.

When you eat a large egg, you gain 6 grams of protein. However, that amount depends on you eating the whole egg. If you separate the yolk from the egg white, then you lose grams of protein.

One of the reasons that choosing to get your protein from eggs is a good choice is because eggs have the essential amino acids that your body needs. You get all of that without getting a lot of calories or fat.

This not only makes eggs a good choice for a meal, but also as a snack. You can snack on a boiled egg and have less calories than you'd get from a prepackaged diet food snack.

Seafood

There are many different types of seafood and there are plenty of ways that you can prepare it. If you fry seafood and load it up with butter or other fatty sauces, then while you'll still get the protein benefit, you'll pile on calories and fat as well.

When preparing seafood, always choose the freshest option and keep the sauces, especially any kinds made with high fat and calories, to a bare minimum if not eliminated completely.

One of the most popular seafood items is tuna. It's simple to make and just as good for you regardless of how it comes packaged. It's extremely low in calories as well as fat - which means that the makeup of this meat is considered to be pure protein.

The protein content of tuna is so high, that's almost all there is to the meat. This is one of the reasons that tuna is often heralded as the best seafood for people who are trying to lose weight.

Consuming just three ounces of tuna at mealtime can give you around 20 grams of protein. But when you look at the calorie content as well, you get less than 100 calories for that serving.

Besides being loaded with protein, tuna is packed with all of the B vitamins that are good for you. It also contains magnesium and potassium - two very important minerals that your body needs plenty of.

And something you might not know about this high protein meat is that it's considered an antioxidant seafood. You can eat this and help give your immune system a boost as well 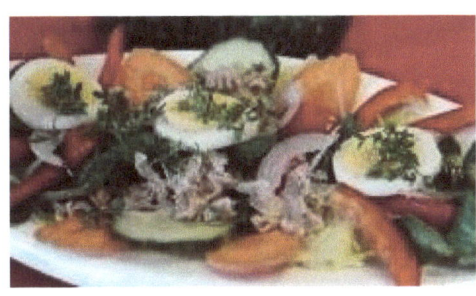 as keep inflammation at bay.

While tuna does have mercury in it, you don't have to worry about this affecting your health. Tuna contains selenium, which counteracts mercury. If you love to eat fish, then you're in luck.

You can lose weight with the high amount of protein found in fish. One type of fish that's a good source of protein is halibut. There are 12 grams of protein for every three ounces of the fish that you eat.

Most portion sizes of this fish are greater than three ounces. When you eat this as a meal, most portion sizes are giving you at least 24 grams or more of protein.

Plus, fish is a great way to get in the amount of omega 3 fatty acids that your body need.

Like tuna, halibut also contains anti-inflammatory properties. It's also loaded with plenty of the B vitamins. Those who enjoy eating fish will love the amount of protein that can be found in tilapia.

Consuming just one fillet of tilapia will give you 23 grams of protein. Plus, it's very low in both fat as well as calories. If you love eating shrimp, that's good news if you're trying to lose weight.

Shrimp can give you almost half of your daily recommended intake of protein. You can get as much as 24 grams of protein from eating shrimp. Just make sure that if you want to have a dipping sauce, you choose a low calorie one.

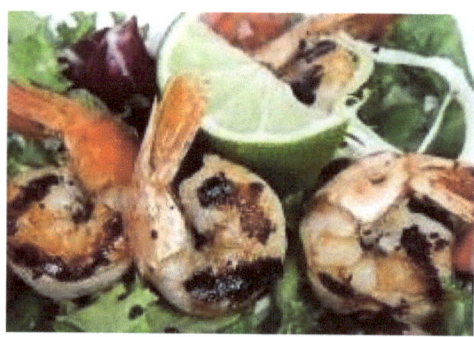

In the seafood family, there are some fish that are so high in protein, they can give you almost a complete days' worth of it. Not only is it beneficial for weight loss but fish is a very tasty form of protein, too.

For a fillet size of just 3 ounces, you can receive up to an amazing 26 grams of protein. Just adding fish to your diet twice a week not only gives you the benefit of omega 3, but it can reduce your risk of heart disease as well.

Fish protein is one of the best kinds of protein to add to your meal planning and it's lower in fat and calories than most other types of meats contain. Just find the type you most enjoy and prepare to cook it in a way that benefits your weight loss goals, such as broiling or grilling.

Top Plant Based Proteins for Your Body

When you're trying to lose weight and you want to eat a diet that has plenty of proteins, you can get the recommended daily amount by adding delicious plant proteins to your meal plan.

Plus, when you eat plant based proteins, you gain a lot in nutrition and health benefits. One of the things that plants can do for you is they lower your cholesterol levels thanks to their fiber content and they can also help prevent many different diseases as well as help those who are currently diagnosed with conditions such as diabetes.

Lentils

Whether or not you're someone who eats meat for protein,

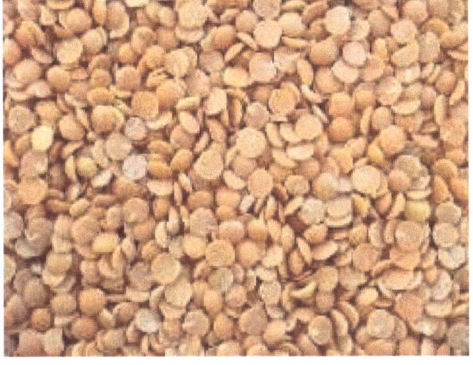

your body can use the additional health boost you gain from eating lentils. While it might seem surprising that these are packed with protein, they are.

In fact, you can gain as much protein from eating a cup of lentils that have been cooked as you can from eating cooked beef. You'll gain an amazing 18 grams of protein for your daily intake amount.

Not to mention that lentils are a superfood when it comes to the amount of iron they can provide for your body. You need iron for your body to be able to make red blood cells.

Without enough, you can feel fatigued. By consuming just one cup of lentils, you get almost 40% of the iron that you need every day. Because the makeup of lentils is a complex carbohydrate rather than mainly a simple carbohydrate, you'll end up feeling fuller longer than if you were to eat other foods with a similar carbohydrate amount.

Plus, lentils are packed with fiber, which helps keep your digestive health in good shape. When trying to lose weight, some people look at the high carb level in lentils and then shy away from them.

But you shouldn't worry because despite this higher carbohydrate level in the food, it's not known to cause your blood glucose to rise. Lentils come in a variety of colors with brown lentils being the ones that you see most often.

The color of the brown with the lentil will depend on the type. So you can get some that are lighter brown while others will be very dark. These are often put into dishes such as soups.

Green lentils can taste a little like green bell peppers or nuts, depending on the color. These kinds of lentils are often served in salad dishes because they can stay firm even after they're cooked.

There are red lentils that come in a variety of colors. This variety, though, doesn't hold onto their firmness after they're cooked. This is one of the reasons that they're most often used in meal planning by adding them to soups or side dishes. These lentils have a sweeter taste than the other varieties.

Edamame

If you've never tried edamame, then you've been missing out. Though the name sounds a little strange, it's a great plant based food that can provide a lot of protein for you as you're trying to lose weight.

Don't let the name fool you. It just means that it's green soybeans. There are different ways that you can eat them or prepare them; all of them are delicious.

This bean packs quite a nutritional punch. When you get a serving size of them, they have an amazing 9 grams of fiber, which help make you feel full so that you're not on the hunt for junk food during the afternoon slump.

If you're thinking that because they're a type of bean, they must be loaded with fat, then think again. A serving size of the edamame has less than 3 grams of fat. They're low in calories, too.

But it's the amount of protein you get in a serving size that's the real weight loss boost. By eating this food, you can add 11 grams of protein to your diet. Not only will you get good fiber and protein benefits, but you'll also be eating a food that nature has packed with vitamins.

Plus, it also has a lot of iron, which your body needs in order to help you on your weight loss journey. This food grows in the pod. The beans inside the pod are very soft.

When you pick or buy them, they can be eaten directly out of the pod - which is the way that a lot of people like to snack on this food. You can purchase these beans already hulled for added convenience.

Besides snacking on the beans straight from the hull, you can add them to various dishes as long as you remove them from the pod since you're not supposed to eat that part of the food.

One of the ways this food is most often served is in salads. You can cook them by boiling the pods or by steaming them, but they don't have to be served warm. Most people also cook them with salt for added flavor.

Hemp Seeds

If you haven't heard of hemp seeds, you're not alone. Many people are unaware of the nutritional power of this protein packed food. At first glance, they do look a lot like sesame seeds, but the taste is a lot stronger.

They're usually used as an add-on ingredient to a dish or as a snack. They're loaded with the power of omega 3 as well as being high in magnesium. They're a great addition to meals for anyone who's trying to lose weight or is looking for better control over their glucose level, since the seeds can be beneficial in that area too.

The seeds are usually hulled and they can be placed in foods like salads or yogurts when you want to add more protein. They can also be lightly toasted and eaten much the same way that you'd eat roasted pumpkin seeds.

A serving size of hemp seeds contains around 11 grams of protein. It's a little higher in fat, so you want to make sure that you're watching the serving size of this food. The seeds are packed with fiber, though, making this a good protein choice.

Quinoa

Quinoa is a food that has a lot of protein per serving. Plus, it's also low in fat. When it comes to giving you energy, quinoa is one of the foods that can definitely do that.

You get a lot of protein for every serving. You can eat a full cup of quinoa and get a little more than 8 grams of protein. Because it's a seed, most people think that it must be loaded with fat, but that's not correct.

This food contains just over 3 grams of fat versus the higher fat content that you'd find in a meat product. Quinoa is rich in vitamins and minerals - including iron, magnesium, vitamin B and fiber.

The fiber content of this food is higher than most other plant based proteins. You'll want to pay attention to your serving size, which is one cup, when eating quinoa because it's one of the higher carbohydrate foods.

It's gluten free and some people use the food just like they would rice when making meals with it. In fact, this food is often used in exchange for meals where some type of grain is called for.

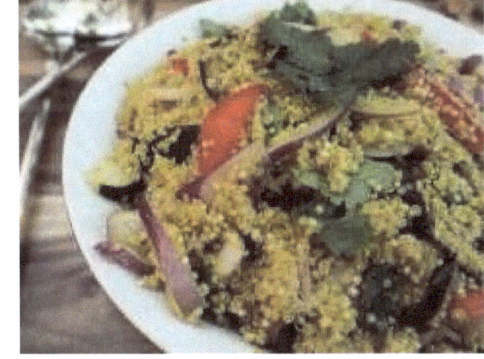

It's one of the most widely chosen foods when dieting because it has all of the amino acids that your body needs. It is considered a superfood. You can choose from black, red or white quinoa and the food contains what's known as flavonoids, which is an antioxidant known to help fight against inflammation, viral illnesses and certain cancers.

It's also known to boost your metabolism, and because it's such a good source of protein, it will help you feel full longer, which can curb your appetite for snacking as well as overeating during meal times.

This food can be added to casseroles so that you get the protein benefit. But it can also be made into pancakes or into meatless burgers. It's a very versatile dish.

Peas

There are some plant foods that will give you as many health benefits as they do grams of protein. Peas are one of those foods. While you might think of peas as just another plant food, it really is a wonderful food to use for both protein and to help boost your weight loss efforts.

While they're loaded with all sorts of health benefits for you, they're not high in fat or calories. Which makes them one of the best plant based proteins that you can use when you're planning out your meals.

Peas have natural nutrients that are known to keep some cancers from occurring. They have the ability to keep your immune system healthy - plus, they help give you plenty of energy thanks to the protein count.

This plant based food is rich in the B vitamins as well as vitamin K, which can work to keep your bones strong and healthy. They're also loaded with antioxidants, which means they can help you fight off illnesses.

They're rich in flavonoids and carotenoids as well. If you're looking for an anti-aging plant food in addition to a food that helps with weight loss, then that's exactly what you've found in peas.

Because peas are so high in fiber, they help keep your glucose levels on an even keel. In turn, that helps keep diabetes at bay. Since the amount of antioxidants in peas is also high, besides eating them for their protein content, peas are great to eat to keep your heart healthy.

Peas contain properties that are known to lower your bad cholesterol level while boosting your good one. Since peas have plenty of fiber, like other plant based proteins, they can keep your digestive system working the way it should.

You can add peas to a salad, soup or other dishes, but you can also eat dried peas as a snack. A serving size of this plant contains 8 grams of protein. It's another versatile option.

Sun-Dried Tomatoes

One of the most often overlooked plants to eat when you want to use protein in weight loss is a sun-dried tomato. It's so packed with vitamins and minerals as well as a healthy serving of protein that it's a plant you can't afford to overlook.

When you dry tomatoes or buy them that way in the store, you'll notice that they taste sweeter. That's only because the water content is now gone and doesn't indicate additional natural sugar content.

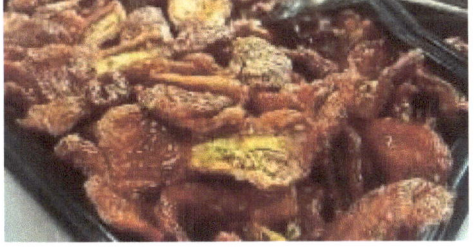

This plant food has over 6 grams of fiber and close to 8 grams of protein. It's a food that's very low in fat, so it's a good choice when you're trying to lose weight. The vitamin and minerals you get in sun-dried tomatoes include iron, potassium, phosphorus and magnesium.

Plus, they're rich in vitamin K, which is needed for bone health. You can use sun-dried tomatoes in a variety of foods including pizza, sandwiches, or salads. It brings many otherwise dull dishes to life.

Chia Seeds

If you've ever seen those Chia Pets, then you've seen the sprouts of the Chia seed. These seeds are filled with benefits for you when it comes to protein and weight loss.

They contain the omega 3 fatty acids and have the power to give you almost 20% of your total calcium requirements. Plus, they contain fiber and are loaded with antioxidants to boost your immunity.

Though they may look tiny, the Chia seeds make up for their size with the amount of protein they can provide just by eating a small amount. If you consume just one ounce of these seeds, you're going to get an amazing 5 grams of protein.

So you can see how you can add these seeds to your diet and easily raise your protein intake. With just that one ounce of seeds, you're also getting 10 grams of fiber.

This amount of fiber in such a little serving size to add to your diet curbs your appetite, helps prevent constipation and gives you energy. The fat content of a serving size is about 8 grams.

Because these seeds are unprocessed, your body can more easily use the nutrients - unlike with some other types of seeds. You can sprinkle the seeds into a main dish, into a cup of yogurt or in your oatmeal and easily get a boost in the amount of protein that you eat.

Using plant based proteins rather than other types of protein options helps you cut calories as well as fat content, which is one of the reasons that people make this switch.

Best Dairy Protein You Can Buy

Some of the foods with the highest amount of protein come from the dairy section of your local grocery store. So if you're someone who enjoys dairy products, you can easily get the amount of protein that your body needs.

Plus, the protein found in dairy products is good for your bones and other areas of your body in promoting good health. It's been proven that dairy doesn't hinder weight loss, either – in fact, it helps you shed pounds.

Why You Should Get Your Proteins from Dairy

Those who advocate cutting out dairy in your diet and avoiding getting your proteins from this food group are wrong. Recent studies have shown that you can't replace the amount of calcium that your body uses on a daily basis with other foods as easily as you can with dairy foods.

If you're a young person in your twenties, then calcium isn't something you really have to worry about as much. The reason for this is because your body is so busy building your bone strength, that it can easily keep up with the calcium that's used by your body.

However, if you're 30 years of age or older, then your body can't keep up production of bone as well as it once did. If you eliminate dairy from your diet, then your bones are left scrambling with a way to get calcium.

So what happens then is that your bones can weaken. They'll fracture and break a lot easier. For those who think they can just up their calcium from other foods, that rarely works.

The reason for that is because you'll have to eat a whole lot more of those other foods to even come close to the amount of calcium found in dairy products. And even then, you won't get the same benefit regardless of how much calcium you eat because your body can't draw in the calcium from those foods as easily as it can from dairy options.

This might help explain why the USDA advocates for people to consume more dairy foods, not less. Dairy products, such as milk, contain a good deal of potassium.

The reason that this ingredient is important has to do with your blood pressure. Most people, even those who are trying to concentrate on using protein to lose weight, have a tendency to still eat foods that have a high sodium content.

This sodium contributes to high blood pressure. Potassium is important in your diet because it gets rid of the sodium and lowers your blood pressure. So when you're trying to lose weight and are looking for good proteins to help with that, make sure that you don't overlook the choices available in the dairy section - especially in milk.

Milk

Milk is an extremely versatile dairy product. It's used in the manufacture of the beverage itself as well as food items as well. So you can drink it or eat products containing it to get the protein that this food has to offer.

Milk comes in a variety of forms. You can buy whole, 2%, 1%, nonfat, evaporated, condensed and even powdered milk. The amount of protein in these products may just surprise you.

If you buy milk in the half gallon or gallon and you choose the 1%, you'll end up getting 8 grams of protein for every 8 ounce cup of it that you drink or use to prepare meals.

If you choose to use 2% milk, you get the same amount of protein. Lowering or raising the fat content of milk doesn't change the protein amount between the two.

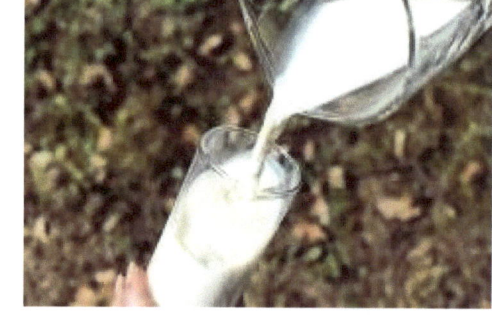

Using milk that's nonfat will also give you 8 grams of protein for every 8 ounce serving. Skim milk also contains the same amount of protein, but gives you fewer calories for each serving that you use.

Evaporated milk contains 9 grams of protein - but that's for only half a cup. So if you use an entire cup of this, then you're getting 18 grams of protein. That seems like a lot of protein just for a milk product, but there are some that contain even more protein than that amount.

Condensed milk is milk where all of the water content has been taken out. It's loaded with vitamins and has an amazing 24 grams of protein for each cup. However, it is extremely high in calories.

Just using one cup of this gives you close to 1,000 calories in your recipes. Powdered milk is a better choice to use if you're going to be making food dishes. This product is even higher in the amount of protein it offers per serving.

You get 34 grams of protein for every cup that you use. Though it's still high in calories, it's not as high as condensed milk. This one has just over 600 calories for every cup that you use.

There is a dairy product that's high in protein that you might not be aware of. It's whey protein. This food is made from separating the whey during the production of cheese. The whey then becomes a powdered protein.

The amount of protein in the product will depend on the brand that you buy. Most whey protein powders usually have at least 20 grams of protein, but many of them have a lot more than that. These products are usually pretty low in calories, depending on which one you buy.

Cheese

Cheese is a milk product that comes in different styles, brands and flavors. You can find mild, sharp and spicy cheeses. The amount of protein in each type of cheese is going to vary as well.

You can easily add to your protein intake by simply switching out a lower protein cheese for one that's higher. Cream cheese is a tasty blend of milk and cream and is used on toast, crackers and in recipes. It has 5 grams of protein for a 3 ounce serving.

Cheddar cheese is one of the most commonly used cheeses on sandwiches. You can have a 1 ounce slice of this and get 7 grams of protein. If you choose to go with American cheese slices, which are also popular, then you only get 5 grams of protein for every slice that you use.

If you choose a slice of provolone instead, you get 7 grams of protein for a slice. Or if you use Swiss cheese, you get 8 grams of protein for every 1 ounce slice that you eat.

Some people like to use Gouda cheese and this kind of cheese also gives you the average 7 grams of protein for the ounce serving size. Parmesan cheese offers 1.9 grams of protein for every tablespoon that's consumed.

Most people eat at least 10-12 grams of this cheese when they use the grated kind on top of a meal such as spaghetti. From there, the amount of protein that you can get from cheese goes much higher.

If you choose to eat a cup of ricotta cheese that's made from whole milk, you'll get 28 grams of protein. When you're preparing a meal, if you use a cup of crumbled feta cheese, you gain 21 grams of protein.

Cottage cheese is a product that's made from soured milk. For people who enjoy eating this dairy product, you can gain 25 grams of protein in just a cup of this type of product.

For years, cheese has developed a bad reputation as being too high in fat - but that's not the case for all types of cheese. While some of them do have a high fat content, not all of them do.

If you eat ricotta cheese, you'll get 32 grams of fat, which is pretty high for a cheese. Most cheese products have between 4-9 grams of fat per serving. If you're concerned about the fat content, choose low fat cheese.

You'll still get a good amount of protein, plus all of the other benefits cheese can give your body. Cheese is packed with calcium and vitamins - including the important B vitamins.

Cultured Dairy Products

There are some dairy products that can give you a good amount of protein that are known as cultured dairy products.

One form of this is the various yogurt products that you can buy.

Yogurt is packed with vitamins and minerals. It contains potassium, calcium, the B vitamins (especially the important B 12 one) and it contains vitamin D. More importantly, many types of yogurt contain probiotics.

If you consume yogurt that has a live, active cultures label on it, it means that the product is providing the good bacteria that your digestive tract needs in order to maintain a healthy balance.

Most regular yogurts have 8 grams of protein for every container of the product. Greek yogurt is a different from regular types of yogurt. In the process of making this kind, the whey is removed.

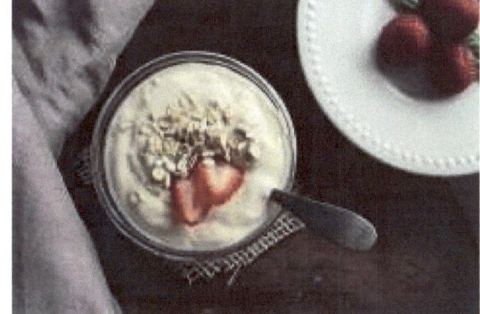

This is one reason that the yogurt is a lot thicker than regular yogurt is. It has more protein per container than regular yogurt does. In fact, Greek yogurt has 17 grams of protein.

But that's not all it has more of. Greek yogurt has more fat than regular yogurt does. So if you want Greek yogurt, but you're watching your fat content, you're going to make sure you want to read the labels and find the one with the lowest amount of fat.

Though it does have a lot more fat than regular yogurt, it does cut down on the amount of sodium that you get. The reason that most people choose Greek yogurt is because it doesn't contain as much sugar as the regular types of yogurt do.

So this means you end up with fewer carbohydrates as well as the additional protein. If you're making recipes that include using sour cream, you can get almost 5 grams of protein for a cup of sour cream.

Using the sour cream that's fat free will give you more grams of protein - with some brands offering 7 grams of protein per cup. If you like to eat dip with your vegetables, that can be a great way to get some additional protein added to your diet.

All you have to do is make the dip using some of the higher protein cheeses shredded and blended with Greek yogurt or even with sour cream, and you've upped your protein count for the day.

Altering your diet to contain a heavier amount of protein than you're used to having takes a bit of strategizing. You need to make sure it's the right kind of protein-carb balance, and space your intake over the course of a day.

But once you get the hang of it, you'll see how much easier it is for your body to rev up its metabolism and burn fat as you shed pounds and reveal layers of lean, taut muscles.

Lose Weight on a Low Carb High Protein Diet

Over the years, eating a low carb diet has grown in popularity, but what many of these low carb diets fail to include is how important it is to make sure that you have a high protein food intake.

Lowering your carbs isn't enough for you to lose weight and keep it off for the long term. That's because carbs and protein actually work together to achieve weight loss success and one without enough of the other simply doesn't work.

The Protein-Carb Myth Busted

The focus of some low carb diets has always been to cut out anything that's above a certain carb level - and that included protein. In fact, some protein foods were put in the "do not eat" category and strategically avoided.

Most people assume that by eating low carb, that they're getting enough of their daily intake of protein. But many people aren't - and that lack of protein is thwarting your weight loss efforts.

The reason you are not losing weight is because you might have thought that by eating protein, you were eating high calorie, fattening foods. Most people don't understand the nature of protein and how the body uses it.

The truth is that protein, while it does contain calories and some fat, isn't high enough in carbs to blow a low carb diet when you're counting calories or carbs.

There are various types of protein that we learned about in this book, so you know which ones to choose for the least amount of carbs.

More than half of all people on a low carb diet don't get the amount of protein that they need. As a result of that, not only is their diet lacking nutritionally, but their health is suffering as well.

Without protein on a low carb diet, you lose energy and you can become sluggish - both physically and mentally. Over half of your calories on a low carb diet should come from protein.

This protein intake should focus on ones that are lean. Instead of getting at least 50-60% of their calorie and carb needs from protein, most people get 15% or less of their carbs and calories from it.

You might think that by eating more of the types of carbs found in meat and increasing your protein level that it will contribute to weight gain, but it's the opposite.

Protein is a weight loss tool. Studies have shown that people whose low carb diets have a strong focus on protein lose weight faster, can prevent or reverse obesity, and also keep other health conditions at bay.

You have to understand what a carb is and how it can contribute to weight gain if you don't make sure that you pair it with protein in your eating plan. But first, you need to take a look at how protein works to get you that lean body you're aiming to have.

How Protein Works

Protein is a weight loss tool unlike any other food. When you focus your meals and snacks on high protein, the protein immediately gets to work in your body to contribute to muscle repair and weight loss.

Protein isn't a food that digests fast. This is one of the reasons that you don't feel as hungry as quickly after having protein. Your body has to make more of an effort to digest protein foods to put them to work for your body.

What that means for you (besides feeling fuller) is that your body is using calories during the digesting process. It's using more effort to digest proteins than any low carb foods or diet foods.

If you need to know how that breaks down into a benefit for you, just take a look at the numbers. Research has shown that people on a low carb diet who add more protein take in about 500 less calories than those who don't up their protein intake.

That equals about 12 pounds of additional weight loss over the course of three months - with you not doing anything except *adding* food. Most people on a low carb diet also add some form of exercise.

They believe it will speed up the weight loss effort. And they're right. But if you're not getting enough protein, you're not losing fat. Instead, what you're losing is muscle mass.

This is why you may have struggled on a low carb diet and been frustrated that you weren't losing enough or gaining lean muscle like you wanted to. Without the amino acids in protein, you won't be building lean muscles.

Low carb foods just don't contain what your body needs. Not only that, but your metabolism will slow down when you don't give your body the right amount of protein.

So if you've been on a low carb diet that's also been pretty low in protein, it's time to make some changes to how you're eating so that you'll see your weight loss kick into higher gear.

It's important that you don't protein load. That means trying to cram all of your protein into one meal. Not only is that not good for you, but you'll be wasting the protein because your body can't use it all at once and protein doesn't store.

Divide the grams of protein you're going to be adding to your eating plan by each meal as well as each snack. This keeps you in protein intake mode throughout the day.

Ad because it digests slowly, it also helps you keep the munchies at bay this way. You have to have protein on a low carb diet from the time you get up to the time you go to bed - and especially after working out.

Study your proteins and make sure that they're packed with all of the amino acids. The best way to make sure of that is by getting your protein from meat. Other proteins don't contain all of the essential amino acids.

If you think that upping your protein intake means you'll constantly be eating chicken or steak and you're thinking you don't have the time or energy to do that, there's an easy way to get the amount of protein that works for you.

You can eat jerky, carry soy nuts or have an energy bar. You can also make a batch of boiled eggs that you can use to take with you when you leave the house to run errands or head to the office.

Final Thoughts

Protein is one of three macronutrients; the other two are fats and carbohydrates. As humans, we need protein to keep our body healthy. It is used to repair and grow tissue, digest and metabolize food, produce antibodies to fight infection, along with being responsible for the production of numerous enzymes and hormones that work to control all of our bodily functions.

But the body has to break down protein into the various amino acids before it can use it. Our body needs 22 different amino acids to function properly. Of those, adults can produce 13 within the body, which are known as non-essential amino acids. The other 9 are essential amino acids and are the ones the body cannot produce. Therefore, we must obtain them from our food, namely from protein.

Foods that contain all 9 essential amino acids are considered complete proteins, while foods only containing some of the 9 are incomplete.

Complete Protein Foods

Most complete protein sources are animal-based and include things like:

- Meat

- Fish

- Dairy products

- Eggs

There are a few plant sources that are also complete, including quinoa, buckwheat, hemp and chia seeds, spirulina and soy.

Incomplete Protein Foods

The rest of the plant-based foods are incomplete either because they lack one or more essential amino acid or the amount they do contain is so low that they can't be labeled as complete. Popular incomplete protein foods include nuts and seeds, legumes, grains and vegetables. And just because a food may be incomplete doesn't make it a bad choice; it just means the food has to be either supplemented with additional protein such as whey powder, or two foods combined to create a complete protein.

Combined Proteins

When two complementary, but incomplete, protein sources are combined, they make a complete protein. Examples include:

- Rice added to various beans or other legumes

- Almonds topped over a spinach salad

- Hummus spread on a whole-grain bread or cracker

- Whole-grain noodles combined with peanut sauce

While the examples suggest two foods are eaten together, they don't have to be. As long as they are consumed the same day, they will function as a complete protein.

Since the body does not store essential amino acids, complete or complementary proteins must be eaten every day in the correct amounts.

How much is enough? Generally speaking, 1/3 gram per pound of body weight. If trying to build muscle through strength training or trying to retain muscle while shredding fat, you may need more – up to as high as 1 gram per pound of body weight.

Protein is the macronutrient we can absolutely not live without. And it is especially important if you are trying to lose weight. Be sure to get your recommended daily amount every day. Without the raw material it needs, our body can't do its job and our health (and weight loss) will suffer as a result.

As a free gift for purchasing this book, I have a free gift for you. It is called **Supplemental Protein Sources - A Guide to Protein Bars, Powder, Shakes and Shakers**. You can download it at:
https://www.dropbox.com/s/4f59of1r6q8x7h5/Supplemental%20Protein%20Sources.pdf?dl=0.

Other Relevant Health Books by This Author

If you would like to read more about losing weight, here is a list of the Createspace links, titles and descriptions:

https://www.createspace.com/4962939

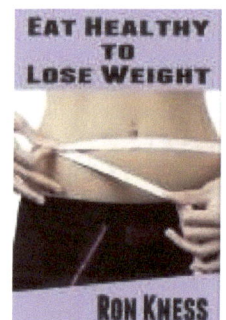

Eat Healthy to Lose Weight

As you read through our book, we show you which foods you should and should not be eating to reach your weight loss goal, along with discussing how to maintain your weight loss and stay within a few pounds of your goal weight. Banish the weight you keep gaining back each time by learning how to live a healthy lifestyle.

https://www.createspace.com/5416348

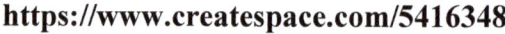

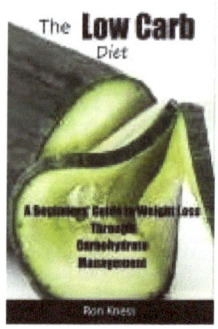

The Low Carb Diet: A Beginner's Guide to Weight Loss Through Carbohydrate Management

In my book "The Low-Carb Diet – A Beginners' Guide to Weight Loss Through Carbohydrate Management", I reveal a successful method of losing weight based in part on the amount and type of carbohydrates you consume.

https://www.createspace.com/6630449

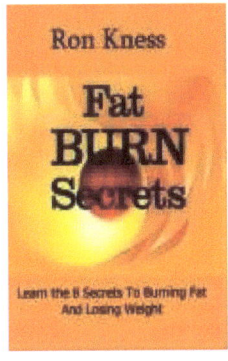

Now you don't have to blindly spend hours of vigorous training and exercise in the gym anymore.

With this blue print for all exercisers out there, you will discover the importance of this amazing combination: making smart food choices in your daily lifestyle and choosing the right work out for your physical endurance.

Follow the easily learnable techniques in Fat Burn Secrets to obtain optimal results and strip that ugly fat off your body, once and for all.

Topics that Fat Burn Secrets covers include:

- Discover the differences between good fats and bad fats. Learn which unhealthy foods with bad fat that you should avoid and strategize a weight loss diet to lose those extra pounds

- Get fit and healthy with the right mindset. Achieving your ideal body shape takes more than just regular exercise and healthy eating. You need to develop a positive and motivated mind set to keep yourself going

- Find out the ninja secrets behind the slim figure of celebrities and apply the successful methods practiced by them to achieve the body that you've always wanted

- Choose the right cardio workout that suits the physical endurance of your body. Combine low intensity and high intensity cardio workout to strip that fat off your body faster

- Lose weight the right way to avoid the yo-yo effect. Be aware of the causes that can lead to this effect so that you won't regain all the fat that you've previously lost

- Practice yoga as a gentle form of exercise and stress management. If you're a beginner and don't know where to start... Perfect. You can learn all the basics with these easy and relaxing poses

- More fat-inducing foods that you should avoid on a regular basis. Fat Burn Secrets will reveal to you why food flavouring like corn syrup and MSG is hazardous to your health

- Are diet supplements recommended for you? Should you take them? Instead of regularly consuming them, why not try out some alternative ways to eating healthier to ensure your body absorbs all the nutrients that it needs

- Detoxification is now becoming a popular trend among dieters to ultimately burn those excess fats. Learn a variety of detox drinks that will surely give your system a good cleanse like never before

- Getting rid of "Love Handles" has always been a challenging feat. But fret not, because with Fat Burn Secrets' step-by-step exercises, you'll be getting rid of these stubborn fats in no time

- And much more to be uncovered in this fantastic game plan!

To sum it up, you'll learn how to:
- Start feeling energetic and be ready to take on the world!

- Crank your metabolic rate up a few notches

- Burn body fat the right way to reveal toned-looking physique hidden beneath layers of unwanted fat

- Get incredibly shapely hips and thighs and lean, toned abs

Get your copy today; start burning fat tomorrow!

About the Author

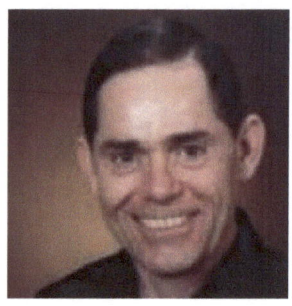

I grew up in Central Minnesota, where my parents owned and operated a fishing resort. Once out of high school I tried a couple of semesters of college, only to quit halfway through the Spring term; I decided at that time that college wasn't for me.

Then I decided to follow my father's previous occupation as an auto mechanic. I graduated from a two-year of vocational training course and worked as a mechanic for five years. While in vocational training, I decided to join the National Guard where I eventually ended up working full-time for 32 years.

So how does all of this relate to writing? In one of my leadership schools, the instructor, who was an English teacher at a juvenile detention center, presented writing to me in a whole new way - a way that started to develop my interest in working with words.

I eventually went back to college on the GI Bill while I was working and earned my Bachelor's degree in Business Administration. Taking a class or two per semester at night and on weekends took me seven years to complete my degree.

Fast forward about 40 years and I now have published over 75 books on Amazon for Kindle, CreateSpace and other publishing platforms.

Besides my own writing, I also ghostwrite ebooks, reports, articles, blogs and do Kindle conversions for clients on a variety of topics.

Today my wife and I are retired from our careers and live in Gold Canyon, AZ. I now write as a retirement business where you'll find me happily sitting in my office typing away on my laptop as I work on my next book or ghostwriting project . . . that is if we are not traveling on a cruise ship - our new-found mode of travel.

www.ingramcontent.com/pod-product-compliance
Lightning Source LLC
Chambersburg PA
CBHW050819290526
45792CB00001B/184